Pharmacology Laboratory Manual
EXPERIMENTAL

Second Edition

VOLUME 1

K.C. Singhal
M.D., Ph.D. (Med.), F.I.A.N., F.I.A.M.S.
Professor
Department of Pharmacology
J.N. Medical College, A.M.U.,
Aligarh - 202 002

CBSPD
CBS Publishers & Distributors Pvt Ltd
New Delhi • Bengaluru • Chennai • Kochi • Kolkata • Lucknow • Mumbai
Hyderabad • Jharkhand • Nagpur • Patna • Pune • Uttarakhand

PHARMACOLOGY
LABORATORY
MANUAL

ISBN: 978-81-239-0554-9

First Edition: 1991
Second Edition: 1997
Reprint: 1999, 2002, 2003, 2004, 2005, 2006, 2007, 2010, 2013, 2016, 2018, 2019, 2023 , **2025**

Published by **Satish Kumar Jain** and produced by **Varun Jain** for

CBS Publishers & Distributors Pvt Ltd
4819/XI Prahlad Street, 24 Ansari Road, Daryaganj, New Delhi 110 002, India.
Ph: 011-23289259, 23266861, 23266867 Website: www.cbspd.com
Fax: 011-23243014 e-mail: delhi@cbspd.com

Corporate Office: 204 FIE, Industrial Area, Patparganj, Delhi 110 092
Ph: 011-4934 4934 Fax: 011-4934 4935; e-mail: publishing@cbspd.com; publicity@cbspd.com

Branches

- **Bengaluru:** Seema House 2975, 17th Cross, KR Road, Banasankari 2nd Stage, Bengaluru 560 070, Karnataka, India
  Ph: +91-80-26771678/79 Fax: +91-80-26771680 e-mail: bangalore@cbspd.com
- **Chennai:** 7, Subbaraya Street, Shenoy Nagar, Chennai 600 030, Tamil Nadu, India
  Ph: +91-44-26680620, 26681266 Fax: +91-44-42032115 e-mail: chennai@cbspd.com
- **Kochi:** 42/1325, 1326, Power House Road, Opp KSEB, Power House, Ernakulum Kochi 682 018, Kerala, India
  Ph: +91-484-4059061-65,67 Fax: +91-484-4059065 e-mail: kochi@cbspd.com
- **Kolkata:** 147, Hind Ceramics Compound, 1st Floor, Nilgunj Road, Belghoria, Kolkata-700056, West Bengal, India
  Ph: +033-25633055, 033-25633056 e-mail: kolkata@cbspd.com
- **Lucknow:** Basement, Khushnuma Complex, 7 Meerabai Marg (Behind Jawahar Bhawan),Lucknow-226001, UP, India
  Ph: +0522-4000032 e-mail: tiwari.lucknow@cbspd.com
- **Mumbai:** PWD Shed, Gala no 25/26, Ramchandra Bhatt Marg, Next to JJ Hospital Gate no. 2, Opp. Union Bank of India, Noorbaug, Mumbai-400009, Maharashtra, India
  Ph: 022-66661880/89 e-mail: mumbai@cbspd.com

Representatives

- Hyderabad 0-9885175004
- Jharkhand 0-9811541605
- Nagpur 0-9421945513
- Patna 0-9334159340
- Pune 0-9623451994
- Uttarakhand 0-9716462459

Printed at Neekunj Print Process, Sonipat, Haryana

PREFACE

There has been a rethinking during the past decade that the syllabus and the method of teaching of pharmacology are at variance with bed side medical practice. It is therefore not surprising that teachers in this discipline are blamed of bothring little to identify the needs of the undergraduate medical student or of not making any serious attempt to revitalize the concept of relevant teaching/ training. Such rethinking has prompted the author to reframe the list of practicals/ demonstrations with the concurrence of teachers from several medical colleges in the country.

The purpose of laboratory techniques in Pharmacology is to develop a scientific foundation for the use of drugs in the prevention, diagnosis and treatment of disease. In these manuals, an attempt has been made to acquaint the undergraduate medical student with the experimental approach to the science of Pharmacology. On the basis of recommendation of Indian Pharmacological Society expert committee for revision of undergraduate curriculum in pharmacology, some conventional practicals which had lost relevance have been deleted and new ones like ADR monitoring, essential drug list, clinical pharmacology experiments, rationale use of drugs, dissolution, disintegration and hardness of tablets have been added.

An attempt is made to give the student an insight into the action of the more important therapeutic agents and to enable him, from the experiments outlined, to grasp the clinical applications of Pharmacology.

The author gratefully acknowledges the help, cooperation and constructive criticism of all the teachers, colleagues and friends in Pharmacology Departments from many medical colleges. Special thanks are due to Dr. Anil Kumar, Dr. Hemant K. Garg and my wife Prof. (Mrs.) Usha Singhal for useful suggestions. Thanks are due to Mr. Subhash Varshney for managing press materials.

1997 **K.C. Singhal**
Aligarh - 202 002
India

Name..

Session..

Class Roll No. ....

Batch ....

Name of the Department & Institution ....

....

....

CERTIFICATE

This is to certify that Mr./Ms...

....has

completed course of practicals in Pharmacy & Clinical

Pharmacology/ Experimental Pharmacology satisfactorily.

Date ....   **Teacher Incharge**

CONTENTS

CENTRAL NERVOUS SYSTEM

DRUGS AFFECTING URINARY OUTPUT

GENERAL INSTRUCTIONS

To make the best of the experiment you must read the theory and the technique of the experiment BEFORE coming to the class.

On the blank sheet provided after the experiment make careful record of the observation and paste kymograph tracings. Honesty with one's self is most important. If observation seems to be wrong consult the teachers so that sources of error may be removed or else have it signed by them, since after all, biological tissues are liable to vary in their response.

Kymograph tracings must be carefully prepared during the experiment. Before varnishing each tracing should be initialled by each partner and also by the teacher incharge with whom you should discuss your records.

Tracings should show (i) the date (ii) the experiment no. (iii) the type of preparation used (iv) the points of application of the drugs (v) temperature of the bath and (vi) the physiological fluid used.

Preservation of tracings

1. All tracings should be rendered permanent by passing through an alcoholic solution of shellac.
2. At the conclusion of the expeiment remove the tracing from the drum by cutting at the seam.
3. Lay the tracing on a flat surface and label with date, name of students and name of experiment. Also indicate the exact position of the writing points when the drug was administered and the amount of drug given.
4. Pass the tracing through the fixing solution provided.
5. Hang the tracing on the rack in the laboratory until dry.
6. Remove the undesirable portion and place the tracing in the note book in the space provided.

Proper use of the drum must be made to obtain tracings and prolong the life of the instruments. When the drum is not in use it should be in the neutral gear and for most experiments it has to run in the slow gear. The speed of the drum for isolated tissues is slower than for heart experiments and has to be adjusted. The drum should move from right to left.

Experiment will often be performed on **live animals** and they are to be treated kindly and handled with care. The teachers will advise you how to handle the various laboratory animals. These directions should be followed explicitly. Improper handling and failure to observe humane technics will be reason for dismissal from the class.

Living tissue with which experiment is to be performed must be handled carefully and as little as possible. Stretching, crushing, drying or otherwise mishandling destroys the cells and it may not be possible to elicit the proper response.

Oxygenation is essential for maintaining the respiration of the tissues. An air connection is provided on every seat for this purpose and this must be properly regulated.

Physiological solutions for different tissues are different. This is of practical importance. A table of solutions used with their compositions are given below.

Table showing compositions of commonly used physiological salt solutions (mg/litre)

Solutions	Glucose	NaCl	KCl	$CaCl_2$	$MgCl_2$	NaH_2PO_4	NaHCO3	Aeration
Frog Ringer	2.0	6.5	0.14	0.12	-	0.005	0.4	Oxygen
Ringer	1.0	9.0	0.42	0.12	-	-	0.5	Oxygen
Tyrode	1.0	8.0	0.2	0.2	$MgSO_4$ $7H_2O$ 0.26	0.5	1.0	Carbogen
Krebs	2.0	6.9	0.36	0.28	0.14	KH_2PO_4 0.16 or NaH_2PO_4 0.11	2.1	Carbogen
De Jalon	0.5	9.0	0.42	0.03	-	-	0.5	Carbogen
Feigan	1.0	9.0	0.42	0.62	-	-	0.6	Carbogen
Locke Ringer	2.0	9.0	0.42	0.24	-	-	0.3	Oxygen
Modified Ringer	1.0	9.0	0.40	0.03	-	-	0.15	Oxygen

Control of temperature : Amphibian tissue will survive for long periods at room temperature. The regular effects can be obtained without using thermostat. Mammalian preparation function best at body temperature and their sensitivity to drugs is often markedly altered by changes in temperature, even as small as 1^0 C. It is therefore essential to use a thermostat.

Recording devices : In most of the experiments the effect which has to be measured is a change in length or tension; in a few it is change in volume, or a change in the rate of flow through the tissue.

Common device for measuring a change in length is a suitable lever.

The length of the lever is usually chosen so as to magnify the response between 5 and 7 fold and the load on the lever is usually between 0.5 g and 1 g. The writing point on the tip of the lever makes a mark on the smoked paper attached to the drum of a kymograph. A permanent record of the experiment is obtained by varnishing the paper.

Two commonly used levers are

1. Side ways writing - the simplist form of lever but it gives a curved line when preparation contracts.
2. Frontal writing - because the point is hinged and the lever writes frontally, it gives a straight line when the preparation contracts.

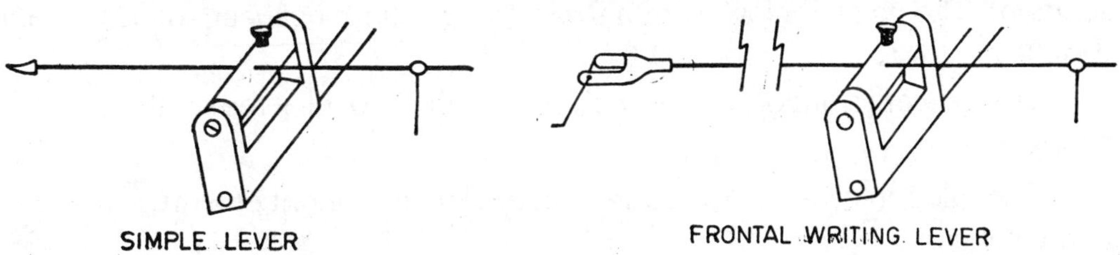

SIMPLE LEVER FRONTAL WRITING LEVER

Stimulators : In a number of experiments it is necessary to stimulate the preparation/animal electrically. The stimulus may vary in duration (milli second), frequency (per second) and strength (volt). Suitable stimulators for producing convulsions in rats or stimulating a nerve are available.

The syringe must be cleaned EVERYTIME a different drug is used.

As regards **human experiments** those of you who are suffering from any infection or have idiosyncracy should consult the teacher before participating.

Bench must remain clean, dry and orderly at all times, it reflects on the method of your working unclealiness will not be tolerated.

List of instruments the students MUST bring in every class

1. A pair of stout pointed scissors.
2. A pair of small thin pointed scissors.
3. A pair of stout forceps.
4. A pair of fine pointed small forceps.
5. A torch.
6. A watch, preferably, with center second hand.
7. A 2 cc all glass syringe with a hypodermic needle No.12.
8. Stethoscope.

Pithing needle, aneurysm needle and bone forceps will be provided on the seats.

Dilution and drugs

Most tissues respond to very small quantities of drugs; usually to a few micrograms (μg), or to a few milligrammes (mg). The weighing of these small amounts is not practicable in these classes. To obtain accurate amount of the drugs used, a suitable quantity is weighed out, using an analytical balance, and then dissolved in a carefully measured volume of the appropriate physiological, solution, e.g. 1.0 g of acetylcholine chloride may be dissolved in 100 ml of Ringer Locke fluid so that 1 ml of the solution will contain 10 mg. By careful volumetric dilution, usually in the ratio of 10 to 1, any desired weight of the drug may be contained in a convenient volume of fluid, 0.1 ml to 1 ml. It is better to refer to the absolute weight of the drug, e.g. 1 μg rather than to say 1 ml of 1 : 1,000,000 solution. The table below summarizes the relation between dilutions and weights.

One percent solution is 1 g dissolved to make 100 ml of the solution (1 : 100 dilution).

The dilution given below contain the following weight of a drug in one ml of the solution.

1 : 100	10 mg per ml	1 ; 20,000	50 μg per ml
1 : 1,000	1 mg per ml (i.e. 1,000 μg per ml)	1 : 50,000	20 μg per ml
1 : 10,000	100 μg per ml	1 ; 2,000,000	0.5 μg per ml
1 : 100,000	10 μg per ml	1 ; 5,000,000	0.2 μg per ml
1 : 1,000,000	1 μg per ml		
1 : 10,000,000	0.1 μg per ml		

Example : If one desires to add 1 ug of a drug to the fluid bathing a tissue, 1.0 ml of a 1 : 1,000,000 solution or 0.1 ml of a 1 : 100,000 solution may be used.

PHARMACOLOGY OF AUTONOMIC NERVOUS SYSTEM

AN OVERVIEW

The autonomic nervous system is also called the visceral, vegetative, or involuntary nervous system. In the periphery, its representation consists of nerves,ganglia, and plexuses that provide the innervation to the heart, blood vessels, glands, other visceral organs, and smooth muscles. It is therefore widely distributed throughout the body and regulates autonomic functions, which occur without concious control.

A clear unerstanding of the anatomy and physiology of the autonomic nervous system is essential to a study of the pharmacology of the autonomic drugs. The actions of an autonomic agent on various organs of the body can often be predicted if the responses to nerve impulses that reach the organs are known.

Table 1 Classification of drugs acting on autonomic nervous system

Autonomic Ganglia		Cholinergic Agonists	Sympathomimetic
Acetylcholine	(a)	**Choline-esters**	**Catecholamines**
Nicotine		Acetylcholine	Adrenaline
DMPP		Methacholine	Noradrenaline
		Carbachol	Dopamine
		Bethanechol	Isoprenaline
	(b)	**Natural alkaloids**	**β–Adrenergic Agonists**
		Muscarine	Isoproterenol
		Pilocapine	Dobutamine
		Arecoline	**Selective β_2-Agonist**
		Oxotremorine	Orceprenaline
		Me N-A-343	Terbutaline
	(c)	**Anticholinesterase**	Salbutamol
		Physostigmine (Eserine)	Ritodrine
		Neostigmine	**α–Adrenergic Agonists**
		Demecarium	Methoxamine

Contd.

Autonomic Ganglia	Cholinergic Agonists	Sympathomimetic
	Diisopropyl phosphoro-fluoridate (DFP)	Phenylephrine
		Mephenteramine
	Echothiophate	Metaraminol
	Isoflurophate	**Selective α_2 Agonists**
		Clonidine (catapres)
		Guanfacine Guanabenz
		α–Methyl dopa
		Miscellaneous agonists
		Amphetamine
		Ephedrine Naphazoline
		Tetrahydrozoline
		Oxymetazoline
		Xylometazoline (Otrivin)
		Pseudoephedrine(Sudafed)

Table 2 Autonomic blocking agents

Ganglion Blocking Agents	Cholinergic Blocking Agents	Adrenergic Blocking Agents
Stimulant	Atropine	**Adrenergic Receptor Antagonists**
Nicotine (Large doses)	Hyoscine	Phenoxybenzamine
Lobeline	Atropine substitutes	(Dibenzyline)
Tetramethylammonium	- Methscopolamine	Phentolamine(Regitine)
DMPP (TMA)	- Methantheline (Banthine)	
Nodepolarizing	- Propantheline	Prazocin (Minipress)
Hexamethonium	(Probanthine)	Ergot alkloids
Pentolinium	- Ipratropium	Indoramin
Trimethophan	- Homatropine	Yohimbine
Mecamylamine	- Cyclopentolate (Cyclogyl)	
	- Tropicamide (Mydriacyl)	
		β-adrenergic Receptor Antagonists
		Non Selective
		Propranolol
		Nadolol Timolol
		Pindolol Labetalol
		Selective β_1 - Antagonists
		Metoprolol Atenolol
		Esmolol Acebutolol

Table 3 Characteristics of subtypes of adrenergic receptors

RECEPTOR	AGONISTS	ANTAGONISTS	TISSUE	RESPONSES	MOLECULAR MECHANISMS
α_1	Adr > NA > Iso	Prazosin	Vascular smooth muscle	Contraction	Stimulation of PLC with formation of IP_3 and DAG; increased cytosolic Ca^{++}
			Genitourinary smooth muscle	Contraction	
			Liver	Glycogenolysis; gluconeogenesis	
			Intestinal smooth muscle	Hyperpolarization and relaxation	Activation of Ca^{++} dependent K^+ channels
			Heart	Increased contractile force : arrhythmias	Inhibition of transient K^+ current
α_2	Adr > NA > Iso Clonidine	Yohimbine	Pancreatic islets (β cells)	Decreased insulin secretion	Inhibition of adenylyl cyclase; activation of K^+ channels
			Platelets	Aggregation	
			Nerve terminals	Decreased release of NA	Inhibition of neuronal Ca^{++} channels
			Vascular smooth muscle	Contraction	Enhanced influx of Ca increased cytosolic Ca

(Contd.)

RECEPTOR	AGONISTS	ANTAGONISTS	TISSUE	RESPONSES	MOLECULAR MECHANISMS
β_1	Iso > Adr = NA Dobutamine	Metoprolol CGP 20712 A	Heart	Increased force and rate of contraction and AV nodal conduction velocity	Activation of adenylyl cyclase and Ca^{++} channels
			Juxtaglomerular cells	Increased renin secretion	
β_2	Iso > Adr = NA Terbutaline	ICI 118551	Smooth muscle (vascular, bronchial, gastrointestinal and genitourinary)	Relaxation	Activation of adenylycyclase
			Skeletal muscle	Glycogenolysis uptake of K^+	
			Liver	Glycogenolysia gluconeogenesis	
β_3	Iso = NA > Epi BRL 37344	ICI 118551 CGP 20712 A	Adipose tissue	Lipolysis	Activation of adenylyl cyclase

Adr = Adrenaline, NA = Noradrenaline, Iso = Isoprenaline

PLC = Phospholipase C IP_3 = Inositol = 1,4,5 Triphosphate DAG = Diacylglycerol

Table 4 Characteristics of subtypes of cholinergic receptors

RECEPTOR	AGONISTS	ANTAGONISTS	TISSUE	RESPONSES	MOLECULAR MECHANISMS
Nicotinic muscle Ach - NM (N_1)	Ach, Nicotine Phenyltrimethyl ammonium (PTMA)	d-tubocurarine α-Bungarotoxin	Neuromuscular junction	End-plate depolarization skeletal muscle contraction	Opening of cationic channel (Na^+, K^+)
Nicotinic Neuronal Ach-NN (N_2)	Ach, Nicotine Dimethylphenyl-piperazinium (DMPP)	Hexomethonium Trimethaphan	- Autonomic ganglia	Depolarization and firing of postaganglionic neuron	Opening of cationic channels (Na^+, K^+, Ca^{++})
			Adrenal medula	Secretion of catecholamines	
			CNS	Excitation or Inhibition	
Muscarinic M_1 Neural	Ach Carbachol Oxotremorine McN-A-343	Atropine Pirenzepine Telenzepine Dicyclomine	Autonomic ganglia	Gastric acid Secretion GI motility	Excitatory Stimulates membrane phospholipase C-Ca^{++} Phosphoinositide system

(Contd.)

RECEPTOR	AGONISTS	ANTAGONISTS	TISSUE	RESPONSES	MOLECULAR MECHANISMS
Muscarinic M_2 Cardiac	Ach Carbachol	Atropine AFD x 116 Gallamine	Heart SA Node	Slowed spontaneous depolarization; hyperpolarization	Activation of K^+ channels inhibition of adenylylcyclase
			Atrium	Shortened duration of action potential; decreased contractile force	
			AV Node	Decreased conduction velocity	
			Ventricle	Slight decrease in contrctile force	
Muscarinic M_3 Glandular	Ach Carbachol	Atropine Hexahydrosila Difenidol	Smooth muscle	Contraction	Similar to M_1
			Secretory glands	Increased secretion	

DRUGS ACTING ON THE HEART

Amongst heart diseases angina pectoris, myocardial infarction, hypertension, congestive cardiac failure and cardiac arrhythmias are the most dreaded but largly preventable and treatable. Coronary arteries get partially or completely blocked in angina and myocardial infarction thus reducing the oxygen supply to the myocardium. Beta adrenergic blockers and calcium channel blockers are clinically useful. β-Blockers have the limitation of being contraindicated in congestive cardiac failure. These group of drugs along with calcium channel blocking, diuretics and angiotensin converting enzyme inhibitors are being commonly employed in the treatment of hypertension. The mainstay for the treatment of congestive cardic failure continues to be digoxin and related cardiac glycosides, besides the use of diuretics, alpha adrenergie blocking agents, arterioles and venous vasodilators and Amrinone an inhibitor of phospho diesterase type III.

Some of the actions of drugs acting on heart can be seen in simple experiments on frog's heart.

Stimulants	**Depressants**
Sympathomimetics	Parasympathomimetics
Adrenaline	Acetylcholine
Ephedrine	Neostigmine
Isoprenaline	
	β-adrenergic blocking agents
Parasympatholytic	Non selective (β_1 & β_2)
Atropine	Propranolol
	Cardioselective
Cardiac glycosides	Metroprolol, Atenolol
e.g. Digoxin	Esmolol, Acebutol
Calcium Chloride	Quinidine, Procainamide
	Disopyramide, Pot.Chloride

EXPERIMENT No. 1

Objective :

To study the effect of cardiac stimulants on frog heart preparation.

Procedure :

1. Fill up the perfusion assembly consisting of reservoir (bulb) rubber tubing, Murphy's drip and the attached venous cannula with the frog's Ringer solution.
2. Pith the frog destroying its brain and the spinal cord.Place it on its back on the board and secure the limbs with the help of elastic bands or pins.
3. Remove the abdominal skin and muscles along the entire length from pelvis to pectoral girdle.
4. Remove the pectoral girdle. Remove the pericardium and expose the heart. Insert a small heart hook, having a thread tied to one end through the ventricular apex. Evert the heart by the thread thus exposing the inferior vena cava.
5. Place a loose ligature in position under the exposed vena cava. Grasp the vessel with a pair of fine curved forceps and cut a longitudinal slit by means of scissors a little below theheart. Insert the cannula connected with perfusion assembly into the slit, directing it towards the heart and tie the ligature tightly. Secure the tubing in position to avoid mechanical disturbance during injection of drugs.
6. Tie the other end of the thread of the heart hook to the recording lever.
7. Run the perfusate from the cannula to the inferior vena cava, then to the right auricle and finally to the ventricle from where it will be expelled out through a silt made in its wall. Adjust the perfusion rate (counted in the Murphy's drip or from the number of bubbles in the reservoir) to 30-35 drop per minute.
8. Record the contractions on a kymograph drum moving at a speed so that 3-4 contractions are recorded per cm. The components of cardiac contractions can be differentiated at faster speed of kymograph drum (see Fig.)
9. Record the following parameters of cardiac contractions.
   (a) *Heart Rate* : It is the number of contractions per minute. In tachycardia

the heart rate is increased and the curves come closer together. The reverse occurs in bradycardia.
(b) *Amplitude* : the height of the curve (Fig.A-B). Increase in amplitude indicates more forceful contraction while decrease, a feebler contraction.
(c) *Tone*: It is the state of partial contraction of muscle at rest. This is denoted by the base line of curves. A rise in base line indicates increase while a fall indicates decrease in tone.

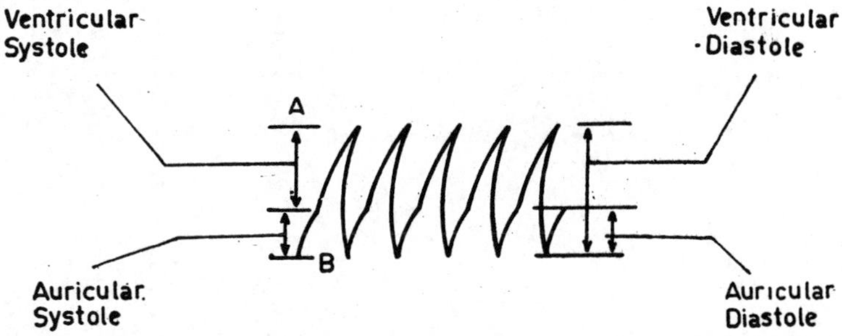

Table 6- Inject 0.5 ml of the drugs in the following order and record the response

	Drug	Solution %
1.	Adrenaline	0.01
2.	Digoxin	0.05
3.	Calcium chloride	0.5
4.	Propranolol	0.2
5.	Adrenaline	0.01
6.	Digoxin	0.05
7.	Calcium chloride	0.5
8.	Calcium chloride 2 ml	0.5

Prescription Writing and Notes

EXPERIMENT No. 2

Objective :

To study the effect of cardiac depressants on frog heart.

Procedure :

1. Mount the frog heart as described in Experiment no. 1 and take the control records on kymograph paper.
2. Inject the following drugs in the order outlined below and study their effects:

S.No.	Drug	Typical Response		
		Amplitude	Rate	Tone
1.	Acetylcholine (0.5 ml of 0.001%) solution	↓↓↓	↓↓	↓
2.	Potassium chloride (0.5 ml of 0.5%) solution	↓↓	↓↓	↓
3.	Atropine (0.5 ml of 0.25%) solution	↑ or—	↑ or—	—
4.	Acetylcholine (0.5 ml of 0.001%) solution	—	—	—
5.	Potassium chloride (0.5 ml of 1%) solution	↓↓	↓↓	↓
6.	Potassium chloride (2 ml of 0.5%) solution	↓↓↓	↓↓↓↓ diastolic arrest	↓↓

Note the change in amplitude, rate and tone of contraction after injection of each drug.

Prescription Writing and Notes

EXPERIMENT No. 3

Objective :

To determine the nature and site of action of an unknown drug on frog heart.

Procedure :

1. Set up the experiment as described earlier. Perfuse heart of frog. Continue perfusion for about 10 minutes, the rate and amplitude of beating heart becomes constant.
2. Elicit the responses of the perfused heart to the administration of
   a) Adrenaline b) Acetylcholine c) $Cacl_2$ d) KCl
3. Inject 0.25 ml of the unknown drug.
   a) If there is chronotropic (increased rate) and / or inotropic (increased amplitude/tone) effect, the drug could be a sympathomimetic amine like adrenaline or a direct stimulant like $CaCl_2$. Adrenergic blocking agent like propranolol can further distinguish between these two categories of stimulants.
   b) If there is inhibition of the heart, the unknown drug could be a cholinergic agent like acetylcholine or a direct depressant. Cholinergic blocking agent atropine can further distinguish between these agents.
   c) If there is no manifest action, inject the four known drugs as before. Refer to the table below for the identification of the cholinergic or adrenergic blocking drugs.

	Adrenaline	Acetylcholine	$CaCl_2$	KCl
Atropine	No effect	Action blocked	No effect	No effect
Propranolol	Action blocked	No effect	No effect	No effect

[18]

Prescription Writing and Notes

DRUGS ACTING ON SMOOTH MUSCLE

Parasympathomimetic drugs like choline esters are capable of producing increase in tone, amplitude of contractions, and peristaltic activity of the stomach and intestine as well as enhanced secretory activity of the gastrointestinal tract. Bethanechol can be of value in certain cases of post-operative abdominal distention and gastric atony and retention or gastroparesis, urinary retention and inadequate emptying of bladder when organic obstruction is absent as in post-operative and post-partum urinary retention and in certain cases of chronic hypotonic, myogenic or neurogenic bladder. Cholinomimetic natural alkaloid pilocarpine is used in the treatment of glaucoma.

Antimuscarinic agents like atropine competitively inhibit the actions of acetylcholine (ACh) on autonomic effectors innervated by postganglionic

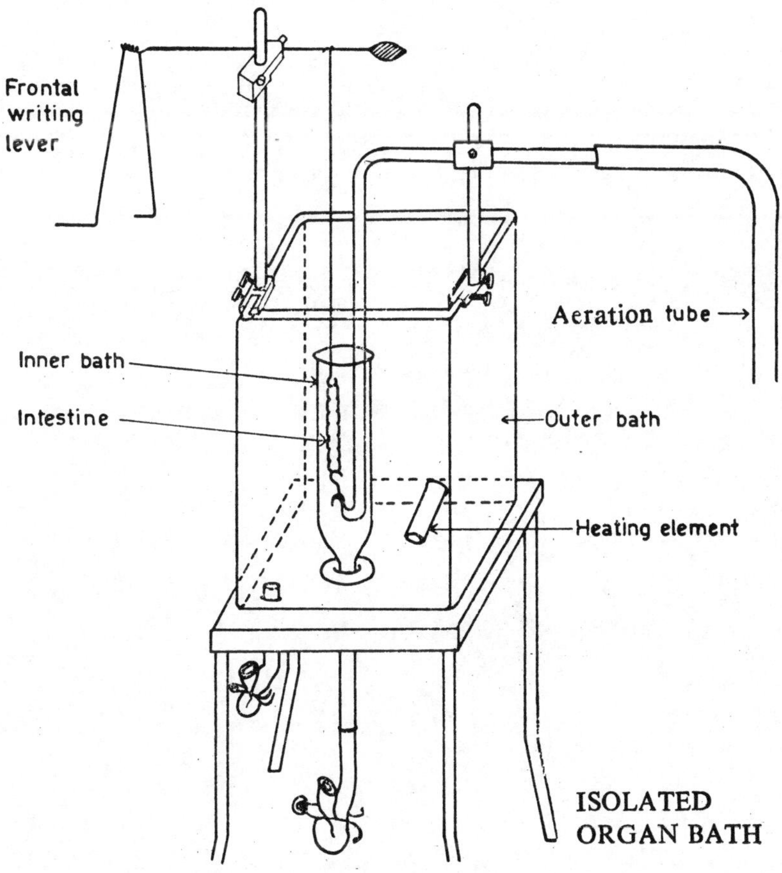

ISOLATED
ORGAN BATH

cholinergic nerves. Therapeutic uses of these agents include (i) to produce mydriasis and cycloplegia (ii) reduce respiratory secretions (iii) treatment of sinus bradycardia (iv) prevention of motion sickness (v) renal and biliary colic and (vi) anticholinesterase and mushroom poisoning. Atropine produce definite and prolonged activity of stomach and intestine characterized by a decrease in tone and in amplitude and frequency of peristaltic contractions.

EXPERIMENT No. 4

Objective :

To study the effect of drugs on the motility of isolated rabbit ileum.

Procedure :

1. Set up Dale's isolated organ bath as shown in figure. Fill the inner bath with tyrode solution and outer chamber with water. Maintain the temperature at 37°C, bath is continuously aerated.
2. Stun a 24 hr fasted rabbit by a hard stroke on the back of neck.
3. Open the abdomen and excise the upper part of small intestine (ileum).
4. Take a piece of about 2 cm in length in a watch glass containing tyrode solution.
5. Flush out the intestinal lumen with the tyrode solution. Remove the attached mesentery and vessels.
6. Handle the tissue very gently.If stretched or handled roughly the response during the experiment may not be proper.
7. Wait till the preparation exhibits spontaneous motility.
8. Anchor one end of the gut to the aeration tube bent U-shaped at one end. Suspend the tube with tissue in 40 ml capacity inner bath and connect the other end with a frontal writing lever so that length of the intestine is recorded.
9. Adjust frontal writing lever in horizontal position, start aeration of the bath and record movements on a smoked slow moving drum.
10. Add drugs in following order, every time a drug is added put a mark near the base line and label appropriately :
    1. Adrenaline 5 μg (0.5 ml of 1 : 100,000)

       Increase or decrease the amount to obtain a suitable response, wash.
    2. Acetylcholine 500 μg (0.5 ml of 0.1% solution)
    3. Atropine 2.5 mg (0.5 ml of 0.5% solution)

       Do not change the bath fluid or repeat the drug.
    4. Acetylcholine same dose as in 2.

       The response to acetylcholine is blocked.
    5. Barium chloride 5 mg (0.5 ml of 1 : 100), wait for 2 minutes.

       Do not change the bath fluid.

       Shifting of baseline indicating increase in tone.
    6. Papavarine hydrochloride 0.5 mg (0.5 ml of 1 : 1000).

Prescription Writing and Notes

EXPERIMENT No. 5

Objective :

To demonstrate stimulant and depressant effects of drugs on rabbit ileum.

To determine, if possible the seat of action of unknown drug.

Procedure :

1. As in experiment No. 4.
2. Record normal movements of rabbit ileum on a slow moving drum.
3. Add unknown drug (0.25 ml). Wait, if no response, add 0.5 ml. If no response increase the drug dose till a definite response is obtained.
4. Observe the tone (base line), amplitude (height of contractions) and frequency of contractions. If any of these three factors is increased the drug is a stimulant. If none of these factors is increased but one or more factors are decreased the drug is a depressant. If the drug is :

Stimulant

Parasympathomimetic
e.g. Acetylcholine
Direct stimulant
e.g. Barium Chloride

- Add Atropine (0.5 ml)
- Wait for 2-3 minutes
- Add unknown drug

No response of unknown drug.
parasympathomimetic
e.g. Acetylcholine

Direct Matching
Acetylcholine

Stimulant effect
of unknown drug
It is probably
direct stimulant
e.g. Barium Chloride

Direct Matching
Add Barium Chloride

Depressant

Sympathomimetic
e.g.Adrenaline
Parasympatholytic
e.g. Atropine
Direct depressant
e.g. Papavarine

Add Acetylcholine (0.5 ml)

No response of
Acetylcholine
unknown drug is
probably
- Parasympatholytic
e.g. Atropine
- Direct depressant
e.g. Papavrine

Add Barium Chloride
(0.5 ml of 1% solution)

Stimulant Effect
unknown drug is
parasympatholytic
e.g. Atropine

No Effect
unknown drug is
depressant
e.g. Papavarine

Stimulant
effect
unknown
drug is likely
to be sympa-
thomimetic
e.g. Atropine

[24]

Prescription Writing and Notes

EXPERIMENT No. 6

Objective :

To differentiate the effect of a sympathomimetic from parasympatholytic drug on rabbit ileum.

Procedure :

1. Carry of out the steps 1-9 of the procedure in Experiment No.4.

2. Add 0.25 ml each of the following drug solutions in the given order.

Adrenaline	0.01%
Acetylcholine	0.1%
Atropine	0.5%
Acetylcholine	0.1%

3. Change the bathing fluid twice or till the normal movements of the gut are restored. Record normal movements.

4. Add 0.25 ml of the following drug solutions in the given order :

Barium chloride	1.0%
Papavarine	0.1%
Acetylcholine	0.1%
Barium chloride	1.0%

Acetylcholine (Parasympathomimetic) augments the movements of the gut by stimulating the muscarinic receptors. Atropine (a natural alkaloid) competitively blocks peripheral muscarinic receptors and is a reversible antagonist of muscarine like drugs. Its effect can usually be overcome if the antagonist concentration is made sufficiently high.

Prescription Writing and Notes

DRUGS ACTING ON SKELETAL MUSCLE

(A) Drugs which facilitate skeletal muscle contraction :

  (i) Acetylcholine. Its deficiency results in a condition called myasthenia gravis.

  (ii) Anticholinesterases neostigmine and pyridostigmine prevent the destruction of acetylcholine and enhance transmission in voluntary and involuntarry muscles, and are used in the treatment of myasthemia gravis.

(B) Drugs which inhibit skeletal muscle contraction are

  (i) Central muscle relaxants.

  Diazepam

  Baclofen

  Dantrolene sodium (has a peripheral site of action)

  (ii) Neuromuscular blocking drugs.

    (a) Non depolarizing (competitive) blockers

    d-tubocurarine

    Gallamine triethiodide

    Alcuronium chloride

    Atrocuricum besylate

    Pancuroneum bromide

    Vencuroneum bromide

    (b) Depolarising (noncompetitive) blockers

    Suxamethonium

(i) Central muscle relaxants

Are used for the relief of muscle spasm or spasticity. They act on central nervous system, with the exception of Dantrolene which has a peripheral site of action.

Diazepam — Oral 2-15 mg in divided doses, max. 60 mg.
IM/IV 10 mg repeated if necessary after 4 hrs.

Baclofen — Oral 5 mg three times a day gradually increased to 100 mg/day.

Dantrolene sodium — Oral 25 mg/day, gradually increased to a maximum of 100 mg 4 times a day.

(ii) Neuromuscular blocking drugs

These drugs by specifically blocking of neuromuscular junction enable light level of anaesthesia to be employed with adequate relaxation of the muscles of abdomen and diaphragm. They also relax the vocal cords and allow the passage of tracheal tube. Patient who have received a muscle relaxant should always have their respiration assisted.

(a) Non depolarising (competitive) blockers:

These drugs cause blockade by competing with acetylcholine at the receptor site at the neuromuscular junction. The action is slower, less complete and of long duration. These drugs should be avoided in myasthenia gravis.

Tubocurarine chloride	20—40 mg IV
Gallamine triethiodide Initially	80—120 mg IV
followed by	20—40 mg as required

Other agents: Alcuronium chloride, Atracurium besylate, pancuronium bromide and vecuronium bromide.

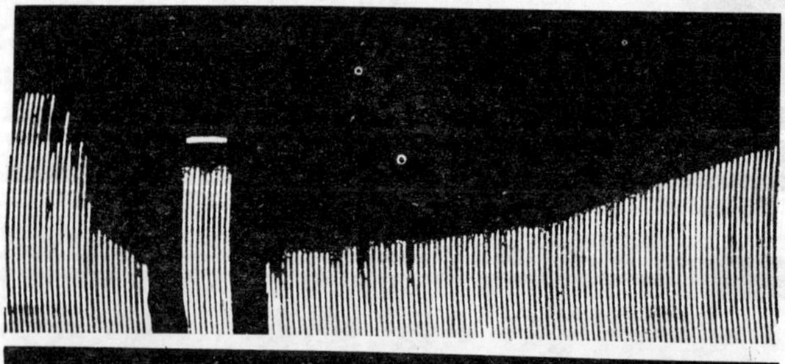

d –TC (150 μg)

CAT TIBIALIS ANTERIOR MUSCLE – NERVE PREPARATION

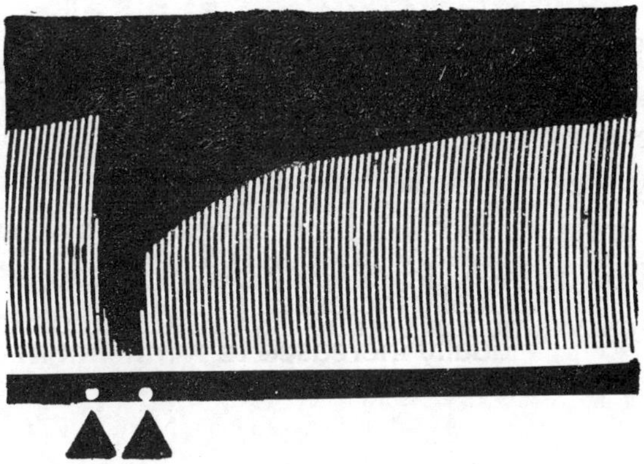

White bar shows **direct muscle** stimulation

(b) Depolarising (non-competitive) blockers:

Suxamethonium is the only drug of this group in use. It mimics the action of acetylcholine at neuromuscular junction and cause blockade. It produces rapid, complete and predictable paralysis, and the recovery is spontaneous. It is usually employed for tracheal intubation.

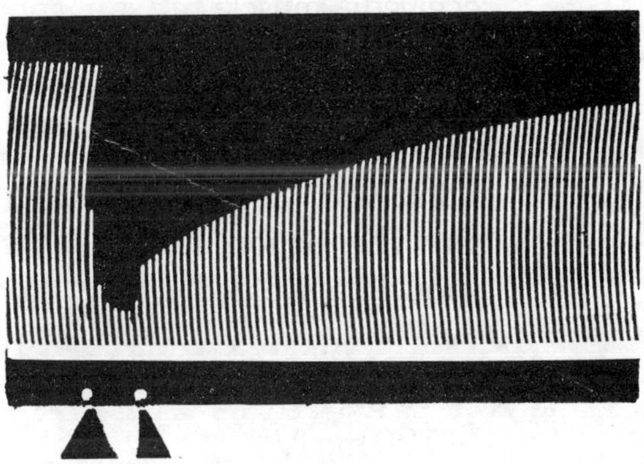

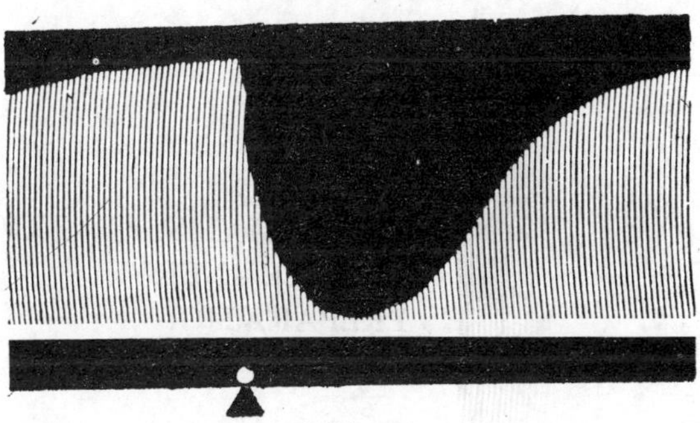

CAT GASTROCNEMIUS SCIATIC NERVE PREPARATION

Dose—20—100 mg IV I. V. infusion—0.1% solution (2-5 ml/minute)

Effect of drugs on skeletal neuromuscular junction

Cholinergic drugs stimulate neuromuscular junction and produce contraction of the muscle. This response is potentiated by anticholinesterases like physostigmine and is blocked by neuromuscular blocking agents like d-tubocurarine. Frog rectus is a voluntary skeletal muscle preparation which shows slow contractions in response to acetylcholine. Nicotinic actions of acetylcholine on skeletal neuromuscular junction can be demonstrated on this preparation.

EXPERIMENT No. 7

Objective :

To demonstrate the stimulant effect of acetylcholine on an isolated frog rectus muscle and its potentiation by anticholinesterases.

Procedure :

1. Set up the Dale's organ bath apparatus as in experiment No. 4
2. Dissect out frog rectus muscle as follows :-

   Pith the frog and remove the skin from the ventral surface of the body. Expose the rectus abdominis muscle. Lift the pelvic end of the muscle with a forcep and carefully separate it from its attachment. Dissect the whole muscle upto and including its attachment to the sternum. Divide the muscle longitudinally.

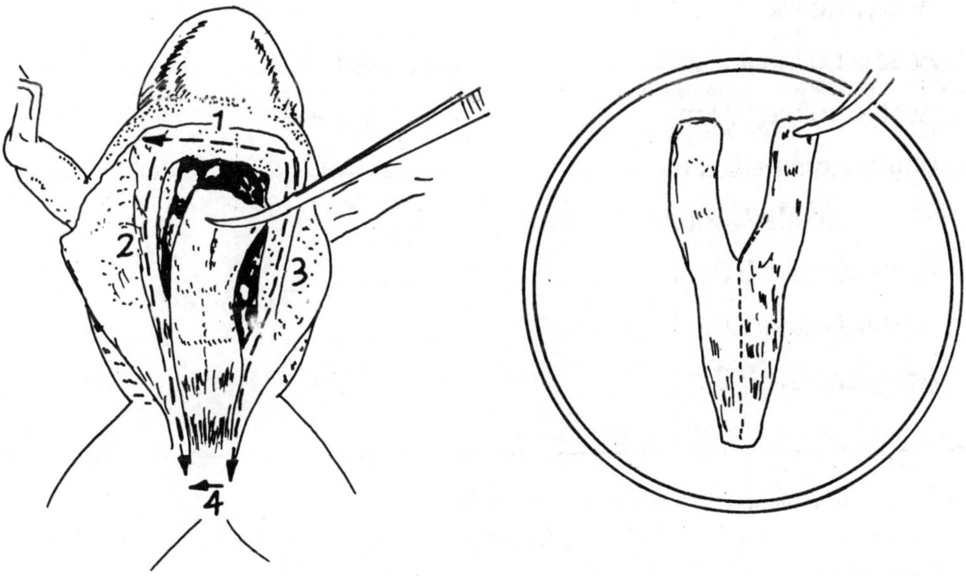

3. Pin the muscle to the board so as to keep it stretched to its normal lenght while it is soaked in frog ringer solution.
4. Sew thread through each end of the muscle.Tie the lower end to the aeration tube, suspend the muscle in isolated organ bath, and tie the thread from the other end to the frontal writing lever.

5. Start aerating the inner bath solution.Aeration should continue throughout the experiment.
6. Record the contractions on a kymograph drum. Allow 20-30 minutes for the preparation to stabilize.
7. Record the reponses to increasing doses of acetylcholine. Allow the muscle to stretch for about 10 minutes by hanging one gram weight on the longer arm of the frontal writing lever in between the responses. Use the doses of drugs as given in table below. Acetylcholine 0.001% solution

Drug	**Response**
Acetylcholine 0.5 ml	+
Acetylcholine 1.0 ml	++
Acetylcholine 2.0 ml	+++
Physostigmine 0.5 ml (0.001% solution)	—
Acetylcholine 0.5 ml	++
Acetylcholine 1.0 ml	+++
Acetylcholine 2.0 ml	+++

+ Stimulation — No response

[33]

Prescription Writing and Notes

[34]

Prescription Writing and Notes

EXPERIMENT No. 8

Objective :

To demonstrate the effect of neuromuscular blocking agent on an isolated frog rectus muscle.

Procedure :

1. Set up the rectus abdominis muscle in an isolated organ bath as described in Experiment No. 7
2. Obtain responses to increasing doses of acetylcholine (0.001% solution).
3. Drain out and refill the bath fluid atleast twice.
4. Add d-tubocurarine 0.01% to the bath fluid. Let it remain in contact with the muscle for 5 minutes. Note the response. Drain out and replace the bath fluid.
5. Obtain responses to increasing doses of acetylcholine (0.001% solution). Note the change in response.
6. Record your observation in table.

Table : Effect of Neuromuscular blocking agent on frog rectus muscle.

Drug	Response
Acetylcholine 0.5 ml	
Acetylcholine 1.0 ml	
d-tubocurarine 0.5 ml	
Acetylcholine 0.5 ml	
Acetylcholine 1.0 ml	
Acetylcholine 0.001% solution	
d-tubocurarine 0.01% Solution	

Prescription Writing and Notes

DRUGS ACTING ON THE EYE

Mydriatics and Miotics

Parasympatholytic agent atropine is a prototype drug used for producing mydriasis (dilatation of pupil) and cycloplegia. Its long lasting action is undesirable for check of refraction. Other parasympatholytic drugs having shorter duration of action, which are commonly used for the purpose, include homatropine, cyclopentolate and tropicamide. To facilitate fundoscopy where only mydriasis is required the sympathomimetic amine phyenylephrine is preferred. Mydriatics (parasympatholytics) must be used with caution, particularly in elderly people, because they raise intraocular tension and may precipitate an attack of glaucoma.

Miotics are employed in ophthalmic practice to constrict the pupil (spreading out the iris as a preliminary to certain surgical operations of the eye) and to lower intraocular tension in various forms of glaucoma. Miotics commonly instilled in the eye as drops include parasympathomimetic pilocarpine, (2-4%), anticholinesterase physostigmine (0.1%).

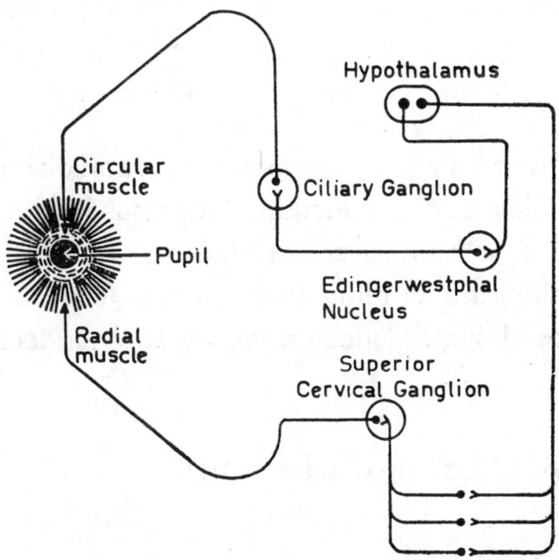

DRUGS USED IN GLAUCOMA

Glaucoma is a condition in which the intraocular pressure is abnormally high. It can result in blindness associated with pressure escavation of optic disc (glaucomatous cupping). The high pressure is attributed to reduced outflow of aqueous, the inflow remaining unaffected.Several group of drugs are used in the treatment of glaucoma.

Miotics

(a) Parasympathomimetic - Pilocarpine hydrochloride 0.5—1% has a duration of action 3-4 hrs.

b. Anticholinesterase - Physostigmine sulphate 0.25 and 0.5%.

Small pupil is unfortunate side effect. Beneficial effect is produced by opening up of the inefficient drainage channels in the trabecular meshwork resulting from contraction or spasm of ciliary muscle. This may also produce spasm of accomodation resulting in blurring of vision and headache.

Adrenergic blocking agents

Timolol maleate	0.25%
Betaxolol HCl	0.5%
Carteolol HCl	1%
Metipranolol	0.1%

Topical application reduces introcular pressure in chronic simple glaucoma, probably by reducing the rate of production of aqueous humour.

Sympathomimetic agent: act both by reducing the rate of production of aqueous humour and increasing the outflow through the trabecular meshwork. Contraindicated in closed angle glaucoma (except when iridectomy has been done).

Adrenaline hydrochloride	1%
Dipirefrine hydrochloride (Prodrug of adrenaline).	0.1%

Mydriatics and cycloplegics

Used for fundosocopy, visual acuity testing, and to provide rest to iris in iridocyclitis.Duration of action in ascending order is given below:

Tropicamide (0.5 and 1%) 3 hours, Cyclopentolate HCI (0.5 and 1%), Hyoscine HBr (0.25%, Homoatropine HBr (1%) all 24 hrs, and Atropine sulphate (1%) 7 days or longer.

Local Anaesthetic : may by used as eye drops for tonometry and removal of foreign body, injected into the eyelids for minor surgery and injected retrobulbar for major eye surgery.

Eye drops

Amethocaine HCL 0.5%, Lignocaine HCL 4%, Oxybuprocaine HCI 0.4% and Proxymetacaine HCL 0.5%.

Prescription Writing and Notes

EXPERIMENT No. 9

Objective :

To study the effect of drugs on (i) the pupil size (ii) the light reflex (iii) the corneal reflex and (iv) the conjunctival blood vessels of rabbit eye.

Procedure :

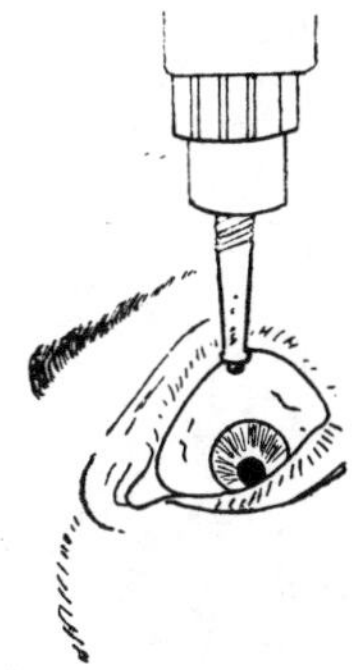

1. Observe carefully, measure (mm ruler) and make sketches showing size of the rabbit pupil in dim light.
2. Test the reaction of the pupil to bright light and note.
3. Instill the drugs into the right eye in the order given in the table. Each drug should be added after atleast 15 minutes of the previous drug. The left eye serves as control. Instill the drug to be tested into the conjunctival sac by means of a dropper. Hold the eye open for about one minute and compress the nasolachrymal duct. Repeat after five munutes if no effect is seen.
4. Note the change in size of pupil - (constriction or dilatation). Sketch the size.
5. Test the light reflex and corneal reflex.

Rabbit No.	Drug	Size of pupil	Light reflex	Corneal reflex	Conjunctival blood vessel
1.	Physostigmine 1% Atropine 1%				
2.	Adrenaline 0.1% Pilocarpine 0.1%				
3.	Atropine 1% Physostigmine 1%				

EXPERIMENT No. 10

Objective :

To measure the intraocular pressure of rabbit eye using tonometry.

LOCAL ANAESTHETICS

Local anaesthesia is the loss of sensation without loss of consciousness, and the central control of vital functions is not impaired.

Local anaesthetics prevent the generation and conduction of nerve impulse. The site of action is the cell membrane and the block is brought about by reduction in membrane permeability to sodium and potassium ions. This would have the effect of stablizing the membrane and reduce its excitability.

Smaller diameter fibers (r) are more easily blocked than large ones (α). There is no vulnerability of motor and sensory fibers of the same diameter. The order of loss of sensation is rather variable but usually pain is abolished first, followed by sensation of cold, warmth, touch, and deep pressure in that order.

Local anaesthetics can be classified into:

Surface anaesthesia : When applied to mucous membrane local anaesthetic agent gets absorbed and makes it insensitive. In this manner conjunctiva, ear drum, nasal mucosa, uretha and larynx can be anaesthetized. Lignocaine 2-4% is used for the purpose.

Infiltration anaesthesia : It is useful for suturing wounds, for circumcision, and for small cysts and lipomas. The anaesthesia takes time. It does not relex abdominal muscles.

Conduction block: It is useful for suturing wounds, for circumcision, and for small cysts and lipomas. The anaesthesia takes time. It does not relex abdominal muscles.

Spinal anaesthesia : In subarachnoid (spinal) anaesthesia local anaesthetic is injected into CSF by lumbar route using lumbar puncture between L 2–3 or L 3–4. Anaesthesia is consistent in the segments it blocks, latent interval is about 10 minutes, duration of action is short (About 2 hr with cinchocaine and 3–4 hr with bupivacaine).

Epidural anaesthesia: The local anaesthetic is injected outside dura (spinal dural pace — thoracic, lumbar or caudal) to anaesthetize spinal nerves as they pass through epidural space. The duration of anaesthesia is longer and can be prolonged indefinitely by using a catheter. But it is less reliable than subarachnoid, has a longer latent interval (about 20 mts.).

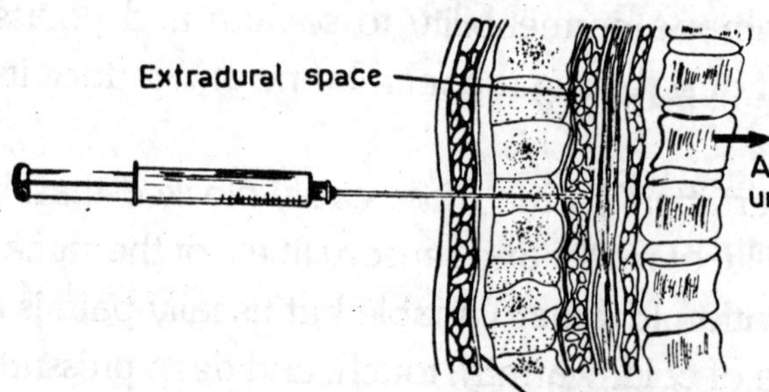

The local anaesthetic used vary widely intheir potency, toxicity, duration of action, stability, solubility in water, and ability to penetrate mucous membrane. These variations determine their suitability for surface, infiltraton, regional, epidural and spinal anaesthesia.

Strength of local anaesthetic agent (%)

Drug	Surface	Infiltration	Regional	Epidural	Spinal
Lignocaine	2–4	0.2–0.5	1	1	5
Procaine	—	0.25–0.5	—	0.5–2	10
Bupivacaine	—	0.25	0.25–0.5	0.5	0.25–0.5

EXPERIMENT No. 11

Objective :

To demonstrate the effect of surface anaesthetics on rabbit cornea.

Procedure :

1. Place a rabbit in a specially designed box or alternatively restrain its movements by wraping in a duster.
2. Clip the eyelashes of both eyes.
3. Elicit winking (corneal) reflex by gently touching the cornea by the tip of a cotton applicator (wick). The wick should be brought from behind to avoid eliciting visual reflex.
4. Expose conjunctival sac by pinching and pulling away the lower eye lid. Instill a few drops of xylocaine 2% in right and procaine 2% in left eye. Close the eyes for a minute by means of pinching together the lower and upper eyelids.
5. Elicit reflex lid reponse (winking reflex) every 5 minutes till reflex is restored.
6. Grade the corneal reflexes as +, ++, +++, and ++++. Record observation in the table.

Local anaesthetic	Time in minutes						
	0	5	10	15	20	25	30
Procaine							
Xylocaine							

Prescription Writing and Notes

EXPERIMENT No. 12

Objective :

To demonstrate the effect of infiltration anaesthesia on rabbit/guinea pig skin.

Procedure :

1. Take a rabbit/guinea pig and clip the hair of the back on either side of the vertebral column and shave two areas of 8 cm diamater
2. Raise 3 equally spaced wheals on both sides of the vertebral column with injection of equal volumes (0.2 ml each) of (i) normal saline (ii) procaine 2% and (iii) xylocaine 3%.
3. Encircle each wheal raised by the injection with ink.
4. Note the pain reaction to ten light pin pricks in each of the sites of injections at intervals of 5 minutes.

   (The number of negative responses (muscle twitch) in each series of pricks gives an indication of the degree of local anaesthesia achieved).
5. Record the responses to pin pricks in each of the wheals in the table.

Number of stimuli eliciting positive responses

Treatment.	Time in minutes						
	0	5	10	15	20	25	30
Normal saline							
Procaine							
Xylocaine							

The sensitivity of the skin is greatest in the midline and slightly more on the front area than on the back area.

Prescription Writing and Notes

BLOOD PRESSURE

Blood pressure is maintained mainly by cardiac output and peripheral vascular resistance. It is controlled by the autonomic nervous system acting on the heart and the vasculature and is consequently affected by cholinergic and adrenergic agonists and antagonists. Drugs that act independently of autonomic innervation on the heart and/or blood vessels would also affect the blood pressure.

Sympathomimetic agents : When adrenaline is injected intravenously into an anaesthetized animal the blood pressure shows an initial increase followed by a fall and then returns to normal (base line). This biphasic response is not seen with noradrenaline which causes only rise in B.P. The rise in blood pressure is due to

1. Action on heart - Positive chronotropic (increase in heart rate) and inotropic (increase in force of contraction) actions.
2. Action on vascular bed - Arteriolar constriction specially in skin, mucous membrane and splanchnic region.

Depressor component of biphasic response of adrenaline is due to effect of adrenaline on β-adrenergic receptors in skeletal muscle blood vessels which dilate. The duration of vasodilator β-effect is longer than vasoconstrictor α-effect.

Dale's vasomotor-reversal phenomenon

This involves blockade of α-adrenergic receptors by an α-adrenergic blocking agent (e.g. Yohimbin, Priscol) to unmask the β-component of the action of adrenaline thus converting the pressor response to a depressor response.

Parasympathomimetic agents

Acetylcholine in a small dose (2 μg) produces a fall in blood pressure due to vasodilatation without any change in heart rate. With a higher dose acetylcholine produces a sharp fall alongwith bradycardia (due to activation of cholinergic receptors in heart)

Nicotinic action of acetylcholine

Acetylcholine acts on two types of receptors, muscarinic and nicotinic. The receptors in vasculature are muscarinic and they mediate the depressor response. They must be blocked by atropine before the nicotinic action (rise in blood pressure) can be demonstrated. The nicotinic response is due to ganglionic stimulation and liberation of adrenaline from the adrenal medulla.

EXPERIMENT No. 13

Objective :

To study the effect of drugs on the blood pressure and respiration of dog.

Procedure:

RECORDING THE BLOOD PRESSURE AND RESPIRATORY MOVEMENTS

1. Weigh the dog. Inject intravenously 30 mg per kg of pentobrabital sodium or 80 mg/kg of 1% chloralose solution (dissolved in warm saline).
2. Cannulate the trachea and connect the tracheal cannula to a recording tembour for recording the respiratory movements.
3. Cannulate the right common carotid artery and connect it through a 3-way cannula to a mercury manometer fitted with a writing lever for recording the blood pressure. Connect the third limb of the cannual to a bottle containing 3.8% citrate solution and fitted with a hand air-pump.
4. Set the 3-way cannula so as to link the manometer to the air-pump. Calibrate the movements of the writing lever by raising the mercury pressure through 0 to 200 mm Hg. at graded intervals, using the pump.

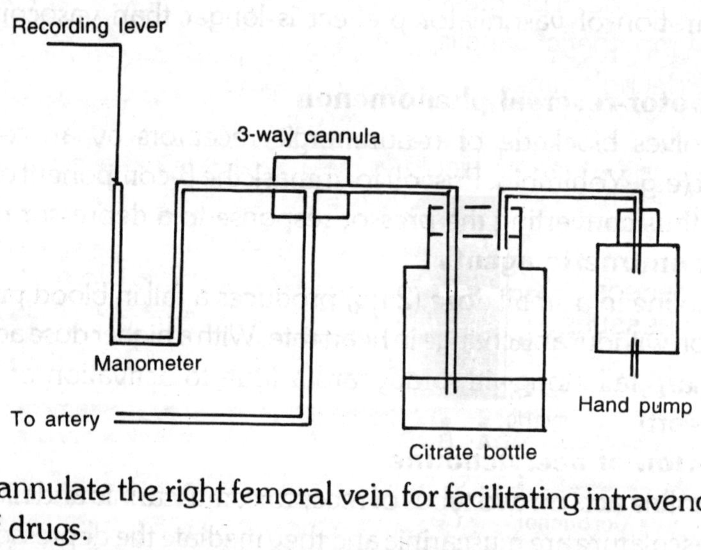

5. Cannulate the right femoral vein for facilitating intravenous infusion of drugs.
6. Start the timer so as to get a time signal at fixed intervals (usually once every 5 seconds).

7. Keeping the pressure in the manometer in the range of the normal mean blood pressure of the dog, turn the 3-way cannula so as to link the artery to the manometer.
If the pressure in the manometer is not kept raised initially, then on connecting it to the artery, blood will flow in the manometer.
8. Start the kymograph and record the blood pressure and respiratory movements. Note the mean blood pressure, heart rate, respiratory rate, the depth (amplitude) and the rhytm of respiration.
RECORDING THE EFFECT OF DRUGS.
9. Record the response of blood pressure and respiration to the intravenous administration of acetylcholine, carbachol and pilocarpine, before and after the administration of atropine 3 mg/kg i.v.).
Acetylcholine, carbachol and pilocarpine, are cholinomimetic drugs. They decrease the blood pressure by acting on muscarinic receptors. Prior administration of atropine which blocks the muscarinic receptors therefore precludes their action.
In higher doses, acetylcholine exhibits nicotinic action characterised by an initial depressor response followed by a long lasting pressor response. The pressor effect is affected through the stimulation of sympathetic ganglia and adrenal medulla with the release of catecholamines.

DOG BLOOD PRESSURE

NICOTINIC ACTION OF ACETYLCHOLINE

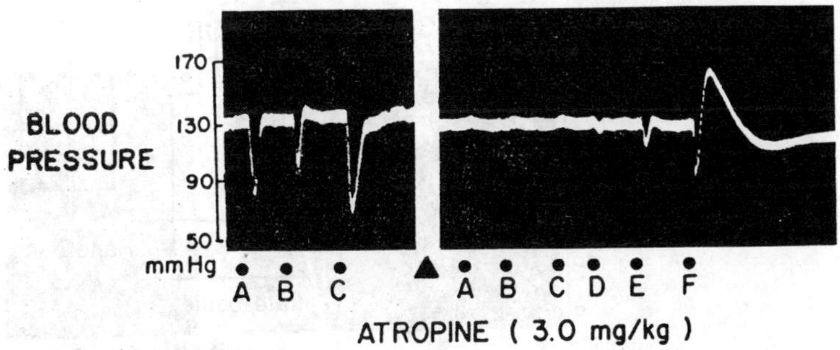

A = Carbachol (0.5 μg/kg) D = Carbachol (0.5 mg/kg)
B = Pilocarpine (5.0 μg/kg). E = Pilocarpine (1.0 mg/kg)
C = Acetylcholine (4.0 μg/kg) F = Acetylcholine (1.0 mg/kg)

10. Record the response of blood pressure and respiration to acetylcholine, carbachol and pilocarpine, before and after the administration of physostigmine.

Physostigmine potentiates acetylcholine by inhibiting true cholinesterase which destroys acetylcholine. It does not affect the efficacy of carbachol (which is destroyed mainly by pseudocholinesterase) and pilocarpine.

DOG BLOOD PRESSURE

POTENTIATION OF ACETYLCHOLINE BY ANTI-CHOLINESTERASE AGENT

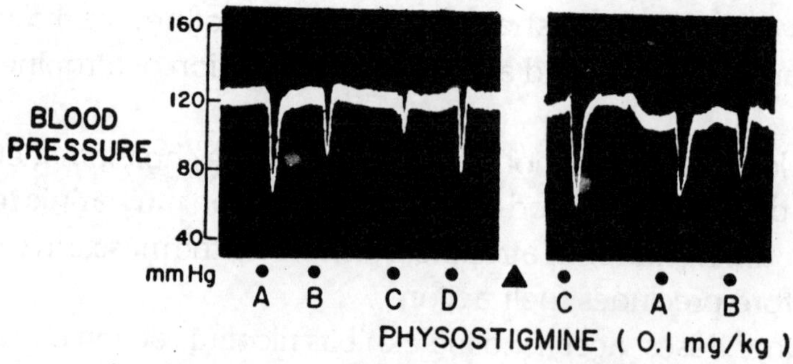

A = Carbachol (0.5 μg/kg) B = Pilocarpine (5.0 μg/kg)
C = Acetylcholine (1.0 μg/kg) D = Acetylcholine (3.0 μg/kg)

11. Record the response of blood pressure and respiration to adrenaline, noradrenaline and isoprenaline before and after the administration of priscol.

alpha- BLOCKADE

DOG BLOOD PRESSURE

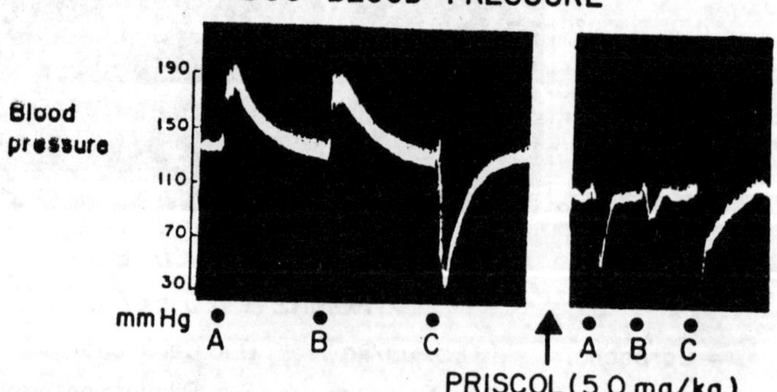

A = Epinephrine (2.0 μg/kg) B = Nor-epinephrine (2.0 μg/kg)
C = Isoprenaline (2.0 μg/kg)

Noradrenaline acts predominantly through α receptors to elevate blood pressure while isoprenaline has a depressor effect, acting mainly through the β receptors ; adrenaline acts though both but has an overall pressor (α) effect.Priscol, an α-adrenergic blocking agent abolishes the pressor effect of noradrenaline but does not affect the action of isoprenaline. It unmasks the depressor (β) effect of adrenaline (known as Dale's phenomenon of vasomotor reversal)

12. Record the response of blood pressure and respiration to adrenaline, noradrenaline and isoprenaline, before and after the administration of propranolol.

Propranolol, a β blocker abolishes the effect of isoprenaline and potentiates the pressor affect of adrenaline but does not effect the action of noradrenaline.

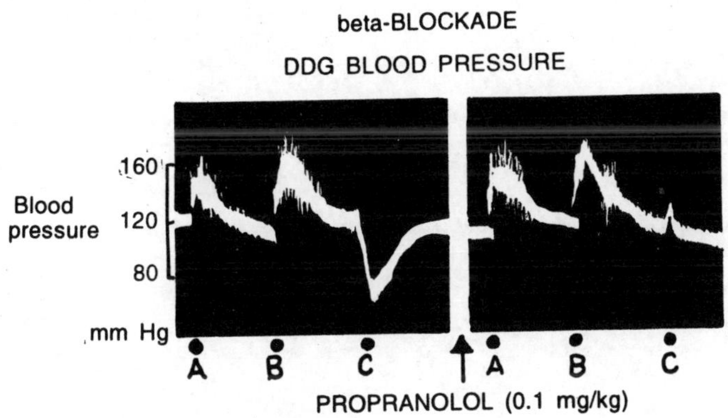

A = Epinephrine (2.0 μg/kg) B = Nor-epinephrine (2.0 μg/kg)
C = Isoprenaline (1.0 μg/kg)

Prescription Writing and Notes

CENTRAL NERVOUS SYSTEM

HYPNOTICS

Except for benzodiazepines (eg. diazepam) hypnotics depress the central nervous system in a relatively non selective, dose dependent fashion, producing progressively calming or drowsiness (sedation), sleep (hypnosis), unconsciousness, surgical anesthesia, coma and fatal depression of respiration and cardiovascular regulation.

A sedative drug decreases activity, moderates excitement and calms the recepient. A hypnotic drug produces drowsiness and facilitates the onset and maintenance of a state of sleep that resembles natural sleep in its EEG characteristics and from which the recepient may be easily aroused.

EXPERIMENT No. 14

Objective :

To study some of the drugs producing sleep and assess their relative potency.

Procedure:

1. Weigh 3 rats and number them.
2. Feed the rats with the following drugs dissolved in water by means of a stomach cannula fitted to a syringe.

	Drug	**Dose**
(i)	Normal saline	
(ii)	Diazepam	0.5 mg / 100 gm.
(iii)	Pentobarbitone	3 mg/100 gm.

3. Assess the hypnotic activity of the drug or the drug combination in terms of loss of Motor activity, Righting reflex, Sound reflex and Pinna reflex. Record the observations, 15, 30 and 45 minutes after drug administration in the following table

Rat	Control Normal saline			Diazepam			Pentobarbitone		
Time	15	30	45	15	30	45	15	30	45
Motor Activity									
1.									
2.									
3.									
Righting Reflex									
1.									
2.									
3.									
Sound Reflex									
1.									
2.									
3.									
Pinna Reflex									
1.									
2.									
3.									

ANTI-EPILEPTIC DRUGS

The terms 'Epilepsy' refers to periodic episodes of disturbed cerebral function that may or may not be accompanied by convulsive movements, loss of consciousness and abnormal behaviour. Several methods have been designed to study potential antiepileptic activity of drugs. These are conducted on animals in which an epilepsy like condition is produced by electrical/chemical stimulation of the brain.

EXPERIMENT No. 15

Objective :

To study the anti-convulsant effect of diphenylhydantoin by supra-maximal electroshock seizure test.

Procedure :

1. Weigh 10 rats and divide them into 2 groups of 5 each.
2. Keep aside one group (Group A) as the control. Administer to the rats in the other group (Group B) diphenylhydantion 30 mg/kg orally by intragastric tube one hour before the experiment.
3. Carefully place corneal electrodes in the eyes of the rats and electroshock (150 m Amp for 0.2 seconds) given with the help of electroconvulsometer. (Electrodes may alternatively be applied on the ear lobes of the animal). Electrodes produce tonic clonic convulsions lasting for about a minute followed by phase of depression characterized by deep inspiration. Rats resume normal activity witin few minutes.
4. Observe the various components of seizures. Note specially the extensor phase of the seizures.

(Antiepileptic drugs useful in the treatment of Grandmal epilepsy abolish the extensor phase of the seizure)

Rat	Control	Diphenylhydantion Treated
1		
2		
3		
4		
5		

EXPERIMENT No. 16

Objective :

To study the analgesic activity of narcotic analgesic by contact heat method (Eddy's hot plate method) in mice/rats.

Procedure:

1. Weigh the mice/rats and number them.
2. Place each mice on a hot plate thermostatically maintained at a temperature of 56.5^{0} C (Alternatively the temperature of the plate can be maintained by placing it on a boiling mixture of equal quantities of acetone and ethyl formate).
3. Note the time between placing of the animal on hot plate and its response to thermal pain (licks, blows paws or dance) is noted as 'Reaction time'.
4. Inject morphine sulphate 15 mg/kg or pentazocine 15 mg/kg intraperitoneally.
5. Determine reaction time again at 20, 40 and 60 min. and record in the table.
6. Mean Reaction Time before and after drug administration is calculated and compared.

Rat/Mice number	Reaction time in seconds			
	control	treated		
		20 min	40 min	60 min
1.				
2.				
3.				
4.				
5.				

This method is useful only for screening of narcotic analgesic. Antipyretic analgesics like acetyl salicylic acid do not modify reaction time to thermal stimuli.

Prescription Writing and Notes

EXPERIMENT No. 17

Objective :

To study the analgesic activity of antipyretic analgesics by chemical stimulus (Writhing Test) in mice.

Aconitine and several chemicals including acetic acid, bradykinin, and NaCl administered intraperitonealy in mice/rat cause irritation and produce within 3 to 10 minutes a writhing or stretching syndrome characterized by a wave of contractions of the abdominal musculature followed by extension of the hind limbs.

Procedure :

1. Weigh the mice, note their weights and divide them into two groups of 5 each.
2. Group A (control) — Inject the mice intraperitoneally with 1 ml/100 g of 10% glacial acetic acid.
3. Record the onset, duration and count the number of writhing in each mice for 30 minutes.
4. Group B(study)—Administer acetyl salicylic acid (aspirin) orally to mice in a dose of 50 mg/kg by stomach tube.
5. After 30 minutes inject glacial acetic acid intraperitoneally (as above).
6. Record the onset duration and count the number of writhings in each mice for 30 minutes.

	Group A Control	Group B–Acetylsalicylic acid treated
Onset (min)		
Duration (min)		
Writhing Count		

Prescription Writing and Notes

EXPERIMENT No. 18

Objecitve:

To estimate the analgesic activity using an analgesio meter (Tail flick method) in rats.

Procedure :

1. Weigh the rats and note their weights.
2. Place the rats in restraining holders so that the tail lies in a groove and protrudes out.
3. Position the holder so that the tail tip is directly over the heated nichrome wire.
4. By adjusting the variac (which regulates the current flowing into the nichrome wire and thereby, its temperature), raise the temperature to a level that gives a tail flick in about 5—6 second.
   In case no tail flick is obtained within 15 seconds due to any reason (eg. an anaesthetic patch on the tail or following drug treatment), discontinue heating. Prolonged exposure to heating may cause skin burns and lead to loss of sensation.
5. Divide the rats into three groups of two each. Administer the following drugs.

Group	Rat Number	Drug
A	1 & 2	No drug - control
B	3 & 4	Morphine hydrochloride 10 mg/kg / Pentazocine 15 mg/kg intraperitoneally
C	5 & 6	Acetylsalicylic acid 40 mg/kg orally

6. Determine the reaction time in seconds of each rat at 15 minute intervals and record it in the table.

Observations :

Rat No.	Reaction time in seconds			
	Minutes after injection			
	15	30	45	60
Control				
1				
2				
Morphine / pentazocine treated				
3				
4				
Acetylsalicylic acid treated				
5				
6				

DRUGS AFFECTING URINARY OUTPUT

DIURETICS

Clinically useful diuretics can be broadly classified into following groups.

1. **Thiazide and related diuretics** - act by inhibiting the renal reabsorption of sodium and chloride at the beginning of the distal convoluted tubule and are moderately potent diuretics. These are used to relieve oedema due to heart failure, and to reduce blood pressure.
2. **Loop diuretics** - inhibit reabsorption from the ascending loop of Henle in the renal tubule and are powerful diuretics. Oral administration is effective within one hour and diuresis is complete within 6 hrs. given intravenously, the action starts within 30 minutes. These are used in pulmonary oedema due to left ventricular failure, in patients with long standing heart failure, oedema and oliguria due to renal failure. Frusemide (lasix), Ethacrynic acid, Bumetanide (Bumet)
3. **Potassium sparing diuretics**-are used in congestive cardiac failure, ascites, nephrotic syndrome and aldosteronism.
   a) Spironolactone (Aldactone, Lactone) competitively inhibits the distal tubular reabsorption of sodium and excretion of potassium that normally occur under the influence of the adrenocortical hormone, aldosterone.
   b) Amiloride and triamterine acts on distal tubule by blocking sodium potassium and hydrogen exchange. Action is weak. These are available in the market as Bidiuret (amiloride + chloro thiazide) and Ditide (triamterine + benzthiazide).
4. **Carbonic anhydrase inhibitor :**

   Acetazolamide (Diamox) is used in the treatment of glaucoma. It inhibits carbonic achydrase, hence reducing the bicarbonate in aqueous humour and the water secreted into it, resulting in a fall in intraocular pressure.
5. **Osmotic diuretics :**

   Osmotic diuretics are pharmacologically inert, resistant to metabolic alteration, freely filterable substances which undergo limited reabsorption by renal tubule. Mannitol is the agent most extensively employed. It is used for prophylaxis of acute renal failure and for the reduction of the pressure and volume of the cerebrospinal fluid.

EXPERIMENT No. 19

Objective:

Estimation of onset, potency, and duration of diuretic action of the following diuretics :

(i) Furosemide, (ii) Hydrochlorthiazide

Procedure :

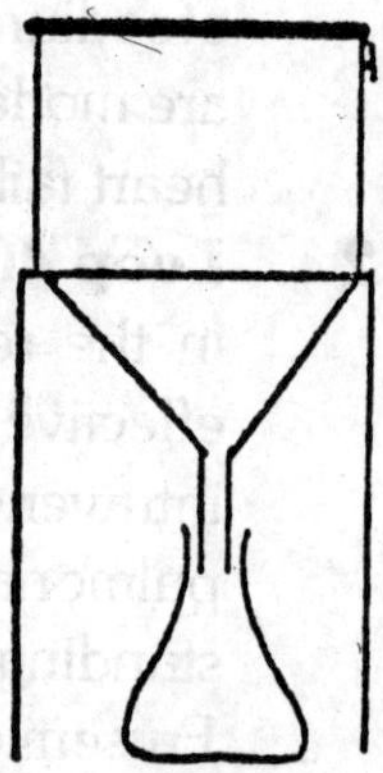

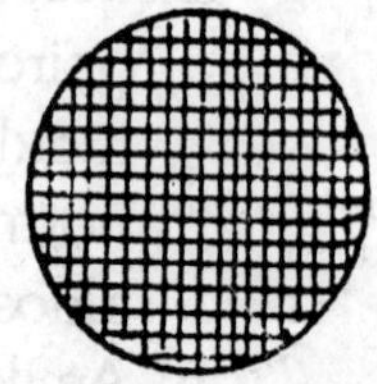

1. Three groups of 4 male rats each, fasted for 18 hours with water and libitum.
2. Weigh each rat and record weight.
   Administer each rat 5 ml/100 gm body weight of a 0.9% sodium chloride by stomach tube or specially designed cannula for this purpose.
3. Group-1 (4 rats) — Place in metabolic cage-control
   Group-2 (4 rats) — Administer Hydrochlorthiazide in a dose of 5 mg/kg body weight orally and place in metabolic cage.
   Group-3 (4 rats) — Administer Furosemide in a dose of 5 mg/kg body weight orally and place in metabolic cage.
4. Measure the amount of urine collected in the flask below each cage at 60 and 90 mts. Take samples for pH and electrolyte estimation.
5. Calculate percent increase in urine volume taking the control volume as 100 percent.

Observations:

Rat No.	Urine Output			
	60 min		90 min	
	ml	pH	ml	pH
Control				
1				
2				
Hydrochlorthiazide treated				
3				
4				
Furosemide treated				
5				
6				